Boba Tea

The Adult and Kid's Guide to boost Energy, Immune System and improve Heart Health with Bubble Tea

Kevin Mary Neo

T a b l e   o f   C o n t e n t s

ISBN: 978-1-63750-105-4

Introduction

Bubble tea first became popular in Taiwan in the 1980s; however, the original inventor is unknown. Larger tapioca pearls were adapted and quickly replaced the tiny pearls. Immediately after, different flavors, especially fruit flavors, became popular. Flavors could be added using powder, pulp, or syrup to oolong, black or green tea extract that is then shaken with ice in a cocktail shaker. The tea mixture is then poured right into a cup using the toppings in it.

Today, there are various available stores that focus on bubble tea. Some cafés use plastic lids, but even more, authentic bubble tea shops serve drinks utilizing a machine to seal the very best in the cup with plastic cellophane. The latter method allows the tea to become shaken within the serving cup and helps it be spill-free until one is preparing to drink it. The cellophane is then pierced with an oversize straw large enough to permit the toppings to feed.

Today, in Taiwan, it is most common for people to refer to the drink as pearl milk tea (*zhēn zhū nǎi chá,* or *zhēn*

năi for short). Even more flavors such as black tea and brown sugar have appeared.

Chapter 1

Bubble Tea

Bubble tea (also called *pearl milk tea, bubble milk tea,* or *boba*) is a Taiwanese tea-based drink invented in the 1980s, that is shaken with ice to produce the *"bubbles,"* a foamy layer with the drink; chewy tapioca balls ("pearls") are added as well. Ice-blended versions are frozen and placed into a blender, producing a slushy consistency. There are numerous types of drinks with an array of flavors. Both most popular varieties are black pearl milk tea and green pearl milk tea.

Bubble teas are categorized into two: *teas (without milk) and milk teas*. Both varieties feature a selection of black, green, or oolong tea, and can be found in many flavors (both fruit and non-fruit). Milk teas include *condensed milk, powdered milk, almond milk, soy milk, coconut milk, 2% milk, skim milk, or fresh milk.*

Some shops offer non-dairy creamer options as well (many milk tea drinks in **THE UNITED STATES** are created with non-dairy creamer). Furthermore, many boba shops sell Asian style smoothies, such as a dairy base and either fruit or fruit-flavoured powder, creating fruity flavours, such as *honeydew, lemon, and so many more (but no tea)*. Now, you will find hot versions offered by most shops as well.

The oldest known bubble tea contains an assortment of *hot Taiwanese black tea, small tapioca pearls, condensed milk, and syrup or honey*. Many variations followed the most frequently are served cold instead of hot. Probably the most prevalent types of tea have changed. The tapioca pearls are produced from the starch from the cassava that was introduced to Taiwan from South USA during Japanese colonial rule.

Bubble tea first became popular in Taiwan in the 1980s; however, the original inventor is unknown. Larger tapioca pearls were adapted and quickly replaced the tiny pearls. Immediately after, different flavors, especially fruit flavors, became popular. Flavors could be added using powder, pulp, or syrup to oolong, black or green tea extract that is then shaken with ice in a cocktail shaker. The tea mixture is then poured right into a cup using the toppings in it.

Today, you can find stores that focus on bubble tea. Some cafés use plastic lids, but even more, authentic bubble tea shops serve drinks utilizing a machine to seal the very best in the cup with plastic cellophane. The latter method allows the tea to become shaken within the serving cup and helps it be spill-free until one is preparing to drink it. The cellophane is then pierced with an oversize straw large enough to permit the toppings to feed. Today, in Taiwan, it is most common for people to refer to the drink as pearl milk tea (*zhēn zhū nǎi chá,* or *zhēn nǎi for short*). Even more flavors such as black tea and brown sugar have appeared.

Variants

Each one of the ingredients of bubble tea can have many variations with regards to the tea store. Typically, various kinds of *black tea, green tea extract, oolong tea, and sometimes white tea are utilized.*

Another variation called yuenyeung (鸳鸯 , named following the Mandarin duck) started in Hong Kong and included black tea, coffee, and milk. Decaffeinated versions of teas are occasionally available once the tea house freshly brews the tea base.

Other types of drink ranges from blended tea drinks. Some could be blended with ice cream. There are also smoothies that contain both tea and fruit.

Although bubble tea started in Taiwan, some bubble tea shops are beginning to add flavors that result from other countries. For instance, hibiscus flowers, saffron, cardamom, and rosewater have become popular.

Tapioca (boba)

Tapioca pearls (boba) will be the prevailing chewy spheres in bubble tea, but an array of other options may be used to add similar texture to the drink. They are usually black because of the brown sugar mixed in using the tapioca. Green pearls possess a little hint of green tea extract flavor. They so are chewier compared to the traditional tapioca balls. White pearls, never to exist confused with the initial pearls, are created with seaweed extract making them slightly healthier but includes an even more crunchy texture.

Jelly will come in different shapes, small cubes, stars, or rectangular strips and flavors such as *coconut jelly, konjac, lychee, grass jelly, mango, coffee, and green tea extract* offered by some shops. Azuki bean or mung bean paste, typical toppings for Taiwanese shaved ice desserts, supply the drinks an extra subtle flavor as well as texture. *Aloe, egg pudding (custard), grass jelly, and sago* are available in most tea houses.

Popping Boba is spheres and also have fruit drinks or syrups within them. Also, they are popular toppings. The countless flavors include *mango, lychee, strawberry, green apple, passion fruit, pomegranate, orange, cantaloupe, blueberry, coffee, chocolate, yogurt, kiwi, peach, banana, lime, cherry, pineapple, red guava, etc.*

Some shops offer milk or cheese foam to fill up the drink too, which includes a thicker consistency similar compared to that of whipped cream. In some instances, the foam is intended to get drunk using the tea by tilting the cup to obtain a good balance rather than mixing the foam into the tea.

Bubble tea cafés will most likely offer drinks without tea or coffee in them. The dairy base for these drinks is flavoring blended with ice, categorized as a snow bubble. All mix-ins that may be put into the bubble tea could be put into these slushie-like drinks. One drawback would be that the coldness with the iced drink could cause the tapioca balls to harden, making it difficult to suck up via a straw and chew. To avoid this from happening, these slushies should be consumed quicker than bubble tea.

Bubble tea stores often give customers the choice of choosing the quantity of ice or sugar, usually using percentages. Bubble tea can be offered in a few restaurants.

History

You will find two competing stories for the foundation of bubble tea. The Hanlin Tea Room of Tainan, Taiwan, claims that it had been invented in 1986 when teahouse owner **Tu Tsong-he** was influenced by white tapioca balls he saw inside the Ya Mu Liao market place. Then made tea utilizing the tapioca balls, leading to the so-called "pearl tea."

Soon after, Hanlin changed the white tapioca balls for the black version, blended with brown sugar or honey, that's seen today. At man\y locations, you can buy both black tapioca balls and white tapioca balls.[citation needed]

The other claim is from your **Chun Shui Tang** tearoom in Taichung, Taiwan. Its founder, Liu Han-Chieh, began serving Chinese tea cold after he observed that coffee was served cold in Japan while on a visit within the 1980s.

The new design of serving tea propelled his business, and multiple chains were established. This expansion began the rapid expansion of bubble tea. The creator of bubble tea is **Lin Hsiu Hui**, the teahouse's product development manager, who randomly poured her fen yuan into the iced tea drink in a conference in 1988. The beverage was well-received in the conference, resulting in its inclusion on the menu. It ultimately became the franchise's top-selling product

The drink became popular generally in most elements of East and Southeast Asia through the 1990s, especially Vietnam.

In Malaysia, the amount of brands selling the beverage is continuing to grow to over 50. The drink is well received by foreign consumers in The United States, specifically around areas with high populations of Chinese and Taiwanese expatriates. Bubble tea includes an extensive existence in the Bay Area, New York, Chicago, along with other large American cities, populated by a lot of those from Chinese and Vietnamese backgrounds. Jollibee, a Filipino junk food chain, once established in Daly City, California in 1998, introduced boba in a broader scale using their semi-discontinued "Pearl Coolers," including the tapioca in popular flavors such as ube and Buko Pandan (coconut).

In contemporary times, bubble tea has achieved cultural significance beyond Taiwan in a few areas for significant East Asian diaspora populations. In America, there's a geographic split with the west coast discussing the drink as *"boba"* as well as the east coast calling it *"bubble tea."*

Health Concerns

In May 2011, a food scandal occurred in Taiwan when DEHP (a chemical plasticizer) was found like a stabilizer in drinks and juice syrups. In June, medical Minister of Malaysia, Liow Tiong Lai, instructed companies selling "Strawberry Syrup", a material found in some bubble teas, to avoid selling them after chemical tests showed these were tainted with DEHP.

In August 2012, scientists through the Technical University of Aachen (RWTH) in Germany analyzed bubble tea samples in a study project to consider allergenic substances. The effect indicated that the merchandise contains styrene, acetophenone, and brominated chemicals, that may negatively affect health. The report was published by the German newspaper ***Rheinische Post*** and caused Taiwan's representative office in Germany to issue a statement saying *"foods in Taiwan are monitored."*

Taiwan's Food and Drug Administration confirmed in September that in another round of tests conducted by German authorities, Taiwanese bubble tea was found to be free from cancer-causing chemicals. The merchandise had also been found to contain no excessive degrees of heavy-metal contaminants or other health-threatening agents.

In May 2013, the Taiwan Food and Drug Administration issued an alert around the detection of maleic acid, an unapproved food additive, in a few foods, including tapioca pearls. The Agri-Food & Veterinary Authority of Singapore conducted its tests and found additional brands of tapioca pearls plus some various other starch-based products bought from Singapore had been similarly affected

In May 2019, around 100 undigested tapioca pearls were within the abdomen of the 14-year-old girl in Zhejiang province, China, after she complained of constipation. However, physicians think that consuming tapioca pearls shouldn't be a concern since it is manufactured out of starch-based cassava root that is easily digested by your body, much like fibre.

In July 2019, Singapore's Mount Alvernia Hospital warned contrary to the sugar content material of bubble tea because the drink had become popular in Singapore lately. Although it recognizes the advantages of drinking green tea extract and black tea in reducing the threat of *coronary disease, diabetes, arthritis, and cancer,* a healthcare facility cautions the addition of other ingredients like non-dairy creamer and toppings within the tea, which raises sugar content of the tea and escalates the threat of chronic diseases. Nondairy creamer is a milk substitute that has trans-fat using hydrogenated palm oil. A healthcare facility warns that fat has been strongly correlated with an elevated risk of heart disease and stroke.

Cultural impact

Within Taiwan

Bubble teas are iconic, to the idea of serving to be a representation of the country. A stylized embossed gold image of bubble tea has been suggested covers for the country's passport alternatively.

Beyond Taiwan

Bubble tea began to rise into popularity in the U.S. because of Congress passing the Immigration and Nationality Act of 1965. This act gave many ethnic groups, specifically Taiwanese immigrants, the capability to immigrate to the U.S. The majority of those immigrants settled down in California, resulting in several bubble tea shops opening around LA. Some of the 1st dedicated bubble tea shops are ***Tapioca Express and Lollicup***. Both of which had been initially owned by Taiwanese immigrants.

Bubble tea is becoming an icon for Asian Americans in LA and is often referred to as simply **"boba"** in California. Even though symbolism, also, has been criticized because of its superficiality and insufficient inclusiveness, it is utilized in the pejorative "boba liberal."

A bubble tea emoji continues to be accepted within the Unicode standard and will be issued in 2020.
Bubble tea can be used to represent Taiwan in the context of the Milk Tea Alliance. From taro milk tea to blended slushies with pudding, we have you covered.
As a person who was raised in what might entirely be the boba capital of America, the San Gabriel Valley milk tea courses through my veins, weekly trips to get boba converted into semi-weekly, then daily. Senior high school study group sessions occurred at boba shops, with Taiwanese-style popcorn chicken and jasmine green tea extract providing sustenance. Debates over which place gets the best, chewiest boba continue steadily to rage, so

when the brand new York Times infamously described boba as *"the blobs in your tea,"* boba enthusiasts across America collectively rolled our eyes.

Boba shops have finally bloomed around America and so are no longer limited by the Taiwanese enclaves they once resided in 15 years back. For individuals who haven't had the opportunity to go through the magic that's boba, and discover themselves staring perplexed on the overwhelming menu filled with customizable choices, this book is here to help you.

Chapter 2

What is Boba?

In simple terminology, it is cassava starch balls.

In explicit terminology, the word boba can holistically, maintain a reference to the complete drink-plus-toppings, typically the most popular topping being tapioca pearls (which also are called boba. I understand it's confusing, but stick with me!). The drink all together is also referred to as *bubble tea, pearl tea, and tapioca tea;* based on what area of the country you're from. As mentioned before, the tapioca pearls, which are also known as "boba," are usually created from cassava starch, a root vegetable from South USA that is generally known as **Yuca**.

Boba the drink in its entirety hails from Taiwan, though its disputed which city and specific shop it started from. Originally, boba pearls were found in shaved ice desserts and paired with syrups, beans, and delectably chewy rice balls. The milk tea was also consumed regularly, and thankfully, someone decided to merge both, thus creating the genius, beloved drink we've today.

Boba culture made its way to America through Taiwanese neighborhoods, and it blossomed near college campuses and high schools, where students would gather for study groups. Most boba shops, nonetheless, are open late and provide affordable snacks and drinks, which made them an ideal quit for late-night hangouts and crunchtime studying.

Bases

The tea base for boba drinks usually is *black or green tea extract* and may be customized with a range of syrups like peach, strawberry, and lychee. Milk may also be put into teas, transforming these to milk teas, and producing for any much creamier, indulgent drink. The classic *"boba milk tea"* order is a black tea with milk and boba.

Some drinks, however, stray from the traditional green and black tea base. Taro milk tea, another big decision, is manufactured out of the tropical taro root. Refreshing fruit teas, often with fruit pieces mixed right in, are often available and frequently caffeine-free. Bright orange Thai tea also makes an appearance of all boba menus, and coffee milk tea is a decision for coffee enthusiasts who would like the very best of both worlds. There are also *oolong, matcha, and white teas* available.

Beyond teas, most boba shops likewise have slushies and milk drinks available too. Slushies are usually created from tea and syrups, which can be thrown in a blender with crushed ice, producing a sweet and frosty treat. Milk drinks have milk like a base, and so are usually sweetened with honey or brown sugar syrup, a beverage that could not sit well for the lactose intolerant.

That said, plenty of boba shops offer milk alternatives like soy, almond, and lactose-free milk, which nicely accommodates the "30 million to 50 million Americans who are lactose intolerant."

Half the fun of venturing out to get boba, that is both a beverage and a snack rolled in a single, is customizing it perfectly for your tastes. Virtually all boba shops provide you with the substitute to adjust the sweetness of the drink, change just how much ice you want, and have even hot and cold options (for if you wish to have your boba fix, but it's freezing outside).

Toppings

Boba

This is the quintessential topping at any tea parlor. Once these balls of cassava root are rolled into bite-size bunches, they're boiled and flavored, often with brown sugar or honey. The effect is a subtly sweet, chewy addition to your drink that escalates the fun of experiencing a milk tea tenfold. If you're trying milk tea for the very first time, I'd recommend going classic and adding boba in your drink.

Pudding

This isn't to become confused with snack pack-style pudding. Pudding at boba shops is custard-like in flavor created from egg yolks, cream, and sugar but firmer because of the addition of gelatin. The closest thing I possibly could compare it to is an incredibly soft flan. They have got the slightest chew and pair nicely with creamier, more indulgent milk teas. Sometimes, boba shops may also possess flavored puddings, like taro or mango pudding. Customize your drink for your preference, as well as add pudding together with boba for different textures!

Grass jelly

Don't worry; it tastes nothing like grass (neither is it created from grass). The treat is manufactured out of Chinese mesona, a plant that's an area of the mint family. The jelly is usually steeped in brown sugar for the slightly sweet, herbaceous taste. Grass jelly comes cut in cubes and texturally is firmer than pudding. I'd recommend pairing grass jelly with any milk tea since it makes an ideal replacement for boba if you feel like experimenting. Also, it goes well with coffee-based drinks.

Aloe Vera

Aloe vera is abundant with antioxidants and reported to be beneficial for your skin layer, why not put it in your drink order? These clear, cubed jellies are soaked inside a syrup and taste refreshing and sweet. As the flavor is a bit subdued, aloe vera jelly goes nicely with bolder, tropical flavors. I'd recommend adding it to citrus drinks, like an orange or passion fruit green tea extract.

Sago/tapioca

Sago tastes like tapioca pudding without the pudding. The texture is chewy and spongy, but a lot more when compared to a tapioca pearl. These delicate, mini pearls make looks in lots of traditional Asian desserts, and pairs nicely with coconut, red bean, and matcha flavors. I would recommend swapping them for boba if you don't need to chew your drink just as much.

Taro balls

Unlike boba pearls, that have a springy texture that bounces back mid-chew, taro balls have a far more gentle melt-in-your-mouth feel to them. These add-ons are produced from taro, mashed with sweet potato flour, and water to create deformed spheres of deliciousness. In Taiwan, taro balls tend to be eaten within a bowl being a dessert, both iced and hot. Add it to your taro milk tea for just a double dose of taro, or pair it with oolong milk tea for your dessert-drink hybrid.

Red bean

If you believe beans don't belong in desserts or drinks, you are passing up on a delicious possibility to have more fibre in what you eat. Red bean (also often called the azuki bean) is usually made by boiling the legume in sugar, producing a fragrant, soft mixture. Traditionally, red bean complements matcha, so I'd recommend having it inside a matcha milk tea for an earthy drink.

Whipped foam/cream

Whipped foam toppings certainly are a recent development in the beautiful world of boba milk teas. Which range from tiramisu crema to sea salt cream, these thick, glossy foams are gently layered together with teas and sipped on delicately. There's even "cheese tea," which is whipped cheese powder or cream cheese that delivers a salty balance towards the lovely syrupy teas of boba shops. The texture is comparable to a fluffy mousse and an incredible foam mustache when enjoyed correctly.

How is it served?

Whenever your boba drink is ordered and customized with ice levels, sweetness, and toppings galore, your creation typically undergoes a particular sealing machine. Boba straws are more significant than typical straws to support the chunks of tapioca, fruit chunks, or other things that you might have within your beverage, and feature a pointed tip to pierce with the covered top of your respective drink (just be sure you own your thumb pressed firmly glaring hole of the straw before you drive it from the film of plastic covering your drink, if not your drink will explode everywhere). Nowadays, there are even metal and glass boba straws available to reduce the necessity for single-use plastic boba straws.

Some boba shops have shorter; stouter cups filled up with their special milk-tea nectars like Half & Half and Honeyboba. Other shops miss the sealing machine and serve their drinks with plastic tops, much like those of drinks at Starbucks. Hot drinks usually can be found in your typical to-go coffee cups, with an attached spoon in case your hot beverage contains toppings.

Whatever container your beverage arrives in, another most sensible thing at boba shops will be the snacks. Boba shops usually offer traditional Taiwanese snacks, which include salty and spicy Taiwanese popcorn chicken, spiced french fries, minced pork with rice, and tea eggs. Larger boba shops may have expanded menus, and extra seating that may change your boba outing from a snack set you back an adequate meal. At those locations, it's unsurprising for the shops to get Taiwanese pork chop, noodles, and dumplings on the menu, with condensed milk-glazed brick toasts for dessert.

What's the price?

Boba milk teas will generally cost you several dollars, based on where you choose your drink. A number of the larger, competent chains like Lollicup and Quickly tend to exist on the cheaper side, with liquors which range from $3-$5, based on the type of toppings you obtain. Toppings usually cost yet another 50 cents per topping; however, they also vary between spot to place.

Tea shops that have a more substantial concentrate on fresh ingredients and organic options, like Boba Guys and 7 leaves, may have slightly higher price points. However, in those cases, you're spending money on quality (tea).

Where Does Boba Tea Result From?

This is a glass or two that started in Taiwan in the 1980s and spread throughout Southeast Asia before finding its way for the U.S. The majority of us think about bubble tea to be synonymous with boba tapioca pearls. Still, bubble tea was originally only a cold milk tea that was shaken until frothy. Sometimes boba was added, but basil seeds or cubes of jelly were also used.

Chapter 3

To Purchase Boba Tapioca Pearls

You'll find boba at nearly every Asian supermarket or online. These marble-sized spheres are produced from tapioca, similar to the smaller pearls we use for tapioca pudding. They can be found in a variety of colors, but all boba experience a reasonably neutral flavor. Once cooked, it's better to mix them with some sugar syrup, thus giving them some sweetness and also helps preserve any pearls you're not using immediately.

Keeping Boba Soft and Chewy

Boba is in their chewiest best if used within a couple of hours of cooking. However, the longer cooking method I outline below helps the boba stay soft and damp for several days if kept refrigerated in simple syrup. They'll gradually begin to harden and be crunchy in the center. For any quick-fix bubble tea, simply boil the boba until they may be soft, 5 to ten minutes.

Putting the Tea in Boba Tea

The sweet and creamy bubble teas you get in the stores are often flavored with special powders and sweetened condensed milk. You can purchase these powders online, combined with the boba themselves. Still, I believe that boba made out of regular tea along with other even more natural sweeteners are simply as good. You only need to produce one glass of strong tea, any tea your choice, and mix it with regular milk, almond milk, sweetened condensed milk, or juice. Just a little simple syrup leftover from soaking the boba helps sweeten things up.

What's your preferred sort of bubble tea?

Measure 2 cups of water for every 1/4 cup of boba. Bring the water to some boil. Bring the boba and stir until they begin floating to the very best of the normal water. Turn heat to medium and cook the boba 12-15 minutes. Remove pan from heat, cover, and allow pearls sit for another 12-15 minutes.

Steps to Make Boba & Bubble Tea

Yield
Makes 1 drink

Ingredients

- ✓ 1/4 cup dried boba tapioca pearls per portion (NOT quick-cooking boba)
- ✓ one to two two tea bags per portion, any kind
- ✓ 1/2 cup water
- ✓ 1/2 cup sugar
- ✓ Milk, almond milk, or sweetened condensed milk
- ✓ Juice or nectar (optional)

Equipments

- ✓ Saucepan
- ✓ Bowl for holding the cooked boba
- ✓ Measuring cups

Directions

Combine the boba with water: Measure 2 cups of water for each 1/4 cup of boba being prepared right into a saucepan. Bring the water into a boil over high temperature. Add the boba and stir gently until they begin floating to the most notable of the water.

Cook the boba: Turn heat to medium and cook the boba for 12 to quarter-hour. Take away the pan from heat, cover, and allow pearls to sit for another 12mins to a quarter-hour.

Prepare the sugar syrup for the boba: As the boba is cooking, get a straightforward sugar syrup to sweeten and preserve them once cooked. Bring 1/2 cup of normal water to some boil over high temperature around the stove or inside the microwave. Remove from heat and stir in 1/2 cup sugar until dissolved. Reserve to cool.

Make a strong cup of tea: This is done either as the boba is cooking or in advance. Allow plenty of time for the tea to cool thoroughly before making the boba. Bring 1 cup of drinking water into a boil. Remove from heat and add the tea bag (or bags); usage one tea bag for regular-strength bubble tea or two for any more robust tea flavor. Take away the tea bag after quarter-hour and chill the tea.

Store the boba until prepared to assemble: After the boba feature finished cooking, drain them from your normal water, and transfer those to a little bowl or container. Pour the sugar syrup over top before boba is submerged. Let sit before boba is room temperature, at least a quarter-hour, or refrigerate until prepared to make use of. Boba is best if used within a couple of hours of cooking, but could be refrigerated for many days. The boba will gradually harden and be crunchy because they sit.

Produce the bubble tea: Pour the prepared tea right into a tall glass and add the boba. Add milk to get a creamy bubble tea, juice for the fruity tea, or leave plain and put in a little spare water. Sweeten to taste with the natural syrup from soaking the boba.

Recipe Notes

Very chilled bubble tea: For an extra-chilly bubble tea, combine all of the tea, milk, and juice, however, not the boba within a cocktail shaker. Put in a few pieces of ice and shake for 20 seconds. Pour right into a tall glass and add the boba.

Shortcut boba: If you'd like immediate gratification, just cook your boba until these are tender, 5 to ten minutes, and use them when they're cool. This sort of boba doesn't stay for long (turning rock-hard in a couple of hours) but is delicious when eaten immediately.

Saving leftover boba and making boba for later: Boba is best if used within a couple of hours of cooking, but could be refrigerated with simple syrup for several days.

The boba will gradually harden and be crunchy because they sit.

How to Drink Boba

Though assorted boba drinks can be found, the most frequent concoction carries a tea base that's coupled with milk or fruit and is usually prepared more than a bed of nice boba pearls. You will find boba milk teas, green teas, black teas, smoothies, coffee drinks, and a slew of other arrangements that may be enhanced with rich flavors that range between lovely to savory. Milk tea is usually prepared with powdered creamers, although fresh milk can be used in a few recipes.

What to know About Boba

The boba pearls give the drink its unique taste and texture. Although pearls could be large or small, the top pearls are most typical in U.S.-based boba cafés.

The tapioca originates from the cassava root, and it is a kind of starch. These pearls are entirely gluten-free and so are commonly blended with brown sugar for flavor, that is how they obtain distinctive black coloring. The texture is comparable to gummy bears, as well as the flavor adapts towards the drink's flavor because the pearls absorb the liquid in the cup.

A Brief History of Boba

Though there are many conflicting stories, boba is mostly thought to have started in Tainan, Taiwan at Hanlin Teahouse. Who owns the teahouse, *Tu Tsong-he*, 1st marketed the drink with white tapioca balls in 1986. Later, he switched for the now-familiar black pearls. By the first 1990s, boba was a sensation throughout East and Southeast Asia. In The United States, it initially became trendy in neighborhoods with predominantly Asian populations and gradually expanded right into a widespread ethnic phenomenon.

Is Boba Healthy?

Much like most coffee and tea drinks, the vitamins and minerals depend on the preparation. Many boba drinks are saturated in sugar, carbs, and calories. If you're worried about your waist or blood sugar levels, you'll want to order a little serving or save this treat for special occasions. Tapioca is without beneficial nutrients alone, but an excellent green tea extract mixture should enable you to circumvent a number of the guilt. Just be aware that an excellent 16-ounce green tea extract boba can pack a lot more than 50 grams of carbs, 40 grams of sugar, and about 240 calories.

Furthermore, a 2012 report done by the University Hospital in Aachen, Germany, discovered that boba might contain trace levels of carcinogens using polychlorinated biphenyls (PCBs). However, some have questioned the results of the analysis because of the researchers' insufficient transparency within their strategy, and as the results haven't been replicated elsewhere. At this time, the findings ought to be taken having a grain of salt-or brown sugar, for example.

While boba may not be the healthiest drink you can choose, it's undoubtedly delicious and worth the casual splurge. Curious to understand a lot more about those mysterious little pearls? Continue reading to see wherever tapioca originates from.

Steps to Make Boba in the Home

Making boba in the home is a superb money-saver, and easy to DIY with only a small number of ingredients. This recipe from your Spruce Eats takes just over one hour from begin to finish.

Total Time: 70 mins

Prep Period: 10 mins

Cook Time: 60 mins

MEAL: 1

Produce the Syrup

Ingredients:

- ✓ 3 parts of water
- ✓ 2 parts white sugar
- ✓ 1 part brown sugar

Gather the ingredients.

- ✓ In a saucepan, bring the water to some boil and add sugars.
- ✓ Decrease the heat and simmer before sugar crystals are dissolved. Remove from heat.
- ✓ Get the Tapioca Pearls

Ingredients:

- ✓ 4 parts water (or even more)
- ✓ 1 part tapioca pearls

Gather the ingredients.

- ✓ Boil water in a big pot. Add the pearls and boil for thirty minutes. Stir occasionally to be sure the pearls aren't sticking to one another or even to the pot.
- ✓ Turn off heat and allow pearls steep within the water for another thirty minutes using the lid on.

- ✓ Drain the tapioca pearls and rinse with cool water to cool them down.
- ✓ Place them inside the sugar syrup. Ensure that the pearls are covered and stir the pearls well.

Help to make the Tea

Ingredients:

- ✓ 3 ounces Tapioca Pearls (from the recipe below)
- ✓ 1 cup brewed tea (cooled)
- ✓ 1 cup milk
- ✓ 4 ice cubes

Gather the ingredients.

- ✓ Place 3 ounces of tapioca pearls in a big glass.
- ✓ Within a cocktail shaker, combine the tea, milk, and ice. Shake well.
- ✓ Pour the shaken mixture into the glass on the tapioca pearls.
- ✓ Serve using a thick straw.

C h a p t e r 4

What's the Vitamins & Minerals of Boba?

If you haven't yet discovered boba tea, be prepared to do this shortly at a teashop in your area. This wildly popular sweetened drink started in Asia. It is a combined mix of sweetened tea, natural or artificial flavors, and a layer of tapioca "pearls" that bob around in the bottom from the cup. The tapioca appears to be bubbles because they come up with the straw, thus the derivation "boba."

Additional names for Boba include bubble tea, pearl milk tea, tapioca tea, ball drink, and pearl shake. The drink is usually served cold, with an extra-wide straw for sucking in the chewy boba together with your drink. Boba tea is ordinarily obtainable in teashops offering extensive menus of flavors and preparations.

What's in Boba Tea?

The word boba tea covers a wide range of special, non-carbonated, non-alcoholic drinks. Most varieties include:

- brewed tea or tea created from concentrate

- milk or perhaps a non-dairy additive to help make the drink creamy
- a lot of sweeteners
- tapioca balls
- Black, jasmine, and green teas are generally used as a base. Many fruit flavors are popular, including mango, kiwi, strawberry, honeydew, and passion fruit.

While there's no "traditional" boba tea recipe, the most natural variety is a sweetened green or black tea with tapioca balls. Nevertheless, you may also get boba tea with no actual boba! Some shops serve boba iced coffee drinks, fruit shakes, and smoothies.

Is Boba Nutritious?

As a way to obtain nutrition, tapioca is a non-starter. Though it is a staple in a few native subsistence diets, its only contribution is as a carbohydrate for quick energy. The vitamin and mineral content material is quite low, and having less fibre is indeed notable that even though you could consume enough tapioca to get some good small nutritional benefit, you'd likely become very constipated. The tapioca balls are produced from tapioca starch or flour, which is extracted through the cassava root, grown primarily in Nigeria and Thailand.

Enjoy boba tea because of its nice, exotic flavor plus the chewy tapioca, not because it's healthy.

The consequences of phenols and polyphenols within tea have already been extensively studied and also have shown promise against cardiovascular conditions and obesity.

However, the amount of sugar you'd consume drinking enough boba tea to get those benefits wouldn't usually be worthwhile. Also, you wouldn't consume enough fruit in the typical boba drink to obtain the advantage of that either. And several teashops employ artificial fruit flavors, or sugary fruit concentrates.

You may get artificially sweetened or unsweetened boba tea, even though the latter is available in several shops and hasn't caught on.

Additive Scares

Within the last couple of years, scandals concerning chemicals put into boba tea mixes with a few manufacturers and imported to America have already been reported. There were reports that *DEHP*, also called *bis(2-Ethylhexyl)phthalate*, may also be used as an additive for tea flavorings. DEHP is a chemical utilized to soften plastics. It had been put into flavorings and mixes to improve color and texture instead of the more costly palm oil. Animal studies have suggested that DEHP causes decreased fertility and growth development issues.

Precaution

While an allergy to tapioca is rare, intolerances towards the ingredient have already been reported, primarily among those people who have celiac disease or other digestive diseases. The cassava root is usually a significant way to obtain carbohydrates using parts of the entire world. Still, improper preparation in the cassava root can lead to significant health symptoms when ingested. For instance, inadequate cooking, soaking, or fermenting with the cassava root or the cassava peel may bring about cyanide poisoning, neurological effects, and goiters.

Some tapioca flours could also contain added sulfite, so boba tea may not be your very best friend when you have a sulfite intolerance.

Essential Information about Boba

Boba, boba milk tea, bubble tea, pearl milk tea: Call it what you would, this sweet drink is more entertainment than nutrients. Enjoy moderation when you are feeling just like a treat, and if you don't possess the intolerances mentioned previously. Drink a cup of green or black tea for his or her unique benefits, and revel in real fruit, not sweetened fruit flavors.

How is Popping Boba Made?

Popping Boba is among the newest & most popular toppings for frozen yoghurt, bubble tea and snow ice. Popping Boba is a distinctive boba that's filled with actual juice flavors that burst in the mouth area. Popping Boba is known as revolutionary in boba technology and maybe the newest topping trend for all sorts of drinks and yogurts alike.

The ingredients for Popping Boba contain *water, sugar, juice, calcium lactate, seaweed extract, malic acid, potassium sorbate, coloring, and fruit flavorings*. The primary ingredient may be the seaweed extract, which is known as to exist the external shell on the Popping Boba. Popping Boba is manufactured out of a popular fresh method of cooking called *"Molecular Gastronomy."*

Molecular gastronomy can be a practice in food science that seeks to research the physical and chemical transformations of things that occur in cooking.

For flavored liquids (such as fruit drinks) containing no calcium, the liquid is thoroughly blended with a small level of powdered sodium alginate, then dripped right into a bowl filled up with a cold solution of calcium chloride.

Just like a teaspoonful of normal water dropped right into a plate of vegetable oil forms just a little bubble of water within the oil, each drop from the alginate liquid will form right into a small sphere inside the calcium solution. Then, throughout a reaction time of a couple of seconds, the calcium solution causes the outer layer of every liquid alginate sphere to create a thin, flexible skin. The resulting *"Popping Boba"* balls are taken off the calcium-containing liquid bath, rinsed inside a plate of ordinary water, taken off the water, and saved for later use in food or beverages.

Boba Everywhere

Bubble tea is not any mere fad. The Taiwan-born drink marrying chewy and sweet tapioca balls with creamy and sweet milk tea, and ice has been around the U.S. for many years, yet its popularity grows. Also called boba for the Chinese slang-derived name in the tapioca balls commonly bought at the bottom with the cup, bubble tea is gaining mouth share and review share since it keeps spreading through the entire U.S. also to new types of businesses.

By "mouth share," boba is on the meteoric rise. "Mouth share" is often a name we used for a metric that tracks the popularity of Yelp of a kind of food or restaurant while controlling for the entire rise in using Yelp. It's the sum of page views for businesses in a confirmed category, divided by all pageviews for food and restaurants - the category's share of most hungry and thirsty mouths likely to Yelp because of their fill.

So far this season, page views for businesses categorized as "bubble tea" in the meals and restaurant categories within the U.S. are up fivefold since 2012, putting the category just before French restaurants and behind ramen. Take into account that the actual growth in traffic to these lenders on Yelp can be a lot more dramatic because overall, Yelp usage has risen. Also, even keeping mouth share unchanged is challenging, as new categories enter the fray all the time. And this analysis isn't including the many businesses that sell boba but aren't categorized as "bubble tea" because of all the other things they do.

In the same way, remarkably, even more Yelpers than ever before can't wait to inform one another about the boba they just drank. The share of reviews in the food or restaurant categories mentioning "boba" is roughly double the share eight years back.

Boba continues to be popular for an extended period, making its continued gains even more impressive. The recent growth in boba's popularity coincides with using the opening or expanding of new boba chains such as Kung Fu Tea and Sharetea, amongst others.

Boba is a nationwide phenomenon: There's a bubble-tea shop Atlanta divorce attorneys state. Some states' residents experienced a bubble-tea option for over ten years; about one-third own gotten their first business categorized as bubble tea recently, including seven within the last six years.

While boba is everywhere, you must go west to get the center on the movement. Among the nation's biggest cities, San Jose and Houston experience the best boba mouth share, accompanied by San Francisco Bay Area and Boston. Boba isn't nearly as big in Miami, Washington, DC, and New Orleans.

Bubble tea isn't just obtainable in boba-focused shops. It's often peddled alongside other drinks. A lot more than one-third of bubble-tea shops will also be classified as coffee and tea, and about as much are classified as juice bars. And nearly one-third are restaurants. Despite boba's Taiwanese roots, Vietnamese may be the most frequent cuisine to become offered by a company selling bubble tea, closely accompanied by Chinese, Asian Fusion, Taiwanese, and Japanese.

Chapter 5

Steps to Make Tapioca Pearls

Producing and using these boba pearls requires two techniques. Initial, you must produce the tapioca pearl 'dough' and form the dried tapioca pearls. Once they are ready, afterwards, you need to cook them before they could be applied in your drink of preference.

THE INGREDIENTS:

- ✓ Flour normal water brown sugar
- ✓ Tapioca flour
- ✓ Brown sugar
- ✓ Hot water

Note: For a far more authentic taste, you can test to get Taiwanese brown sugar ('black sugar'). However, if you're struggling to find this, then any darkish sugar will continue to work.

Needed to get the Brown Sugar Boba Drink

Extra brown sugar

Your favorite tea/iced tea, flavored milk as well as juice/smoothie (I used Bantha Milk - all-natural blue milk).

Diy Tapioca Pearls (Boba) How-To:

Start by warming up water and sugar inside a medium-sized pot, and heat to medium. Stir until all of the sugar has dissolved. Then switch off the heat.

Bring about one tablespoon from the tapioca flour and stir until well combined. Make sure you will find no lumps. Then turn the heat on again and stir the mixture until it starts thickening.

Steps to make Tapioca dough for Tapioca pearls 'boba pearls'

- ✓ Once it becomes thick, remove from heat. Add all of those other tapioca flour and mix well until you have a sticky dough.
- ✓ On the lightly floured surface (floured with tapioca flour), knead the dough until it becomes uniform, soft and elastic. Tapioca dough can be quite sticky, so then add extra flour, if needed.

- ✓ While rolling the dough, if it's far more convenient to utilize 1 / 2 of it at the same time, be sure to cover the spouse, so that it doesn't dry.
- ✓ Roll the dough into thin long rod-like pieces. Each roll must become quite thin, as the tapioca pearls will expand when cooked down the road.
- ✓ Slice the rolls into small pieces. Then roll each piece right into a tiny ball. Repeat with all of that other dough. Now, you might have your dried tapioca pearls ready.

Note: If you wish to speed up this technique, you can miss rolling them into balls altogether. The 'cube' like shapes you'll have may not be as pretty, but they'll taste the same (just make sure they're as even in dimensions as you possibly can, when cutting).

How to Store Un-Cooked Tapioca Pearls:

If you're not thinking about building your bubble tea immediately, or you've made an enormous batch in the boba, then these could be stored for later use. You don't need to refrigerate them simply retain in an airtight container within a cool, dry area, and they are ready to be utilized for six months.

If you do store them inside the fridge, this may affect the texture with the boba and get them to just a little harder - although they'll be fine to utilize.

You can even freeze the dough as well as the cooked pearls, which is thought to keep up with the texture. If freezing the dough, after that, you can boil them immediately without waiting to allow them to thaw.

How to Cook Tapioca Pearls

In a big saucepan, boil enough water to protect your boba. Then add the tapioca pearls for the boiling water (carefully, and that means you don't splash yourself). Stir well, so they don't stick to the bottom on the pot or each other. Encompass the pot. Boil for 20 minutes, then let them rest for another 20 minutes.

Finally, drain the boba.

Now you can either add these to your favorite tea or milk drink or first make a sugar syrup for an extra special treat. I suggest choosing the extra next thing, though, as this takes the pearls from being 'nice' to 'more please' adding a caramel-like flavor, and softening the texture.

DIY Brown Sugar Boba Drink

To help make the brown sugar tapioca peals, first warm-up the brown sugar over medium heat for two minutes. The sugar only must be heated up, not completely melted. Add the boba and stir well to coat all of the pearls using the sugar.

Steps to Make Bubble Milk Tea

For a typical boba, a black tea base may be the norm. However, you can even use several herbal teas, flavored milk, as well as juices/smoothies as your drink base.

When developing a tea then simply steep the tea bags/tea leaves in warm milk (alternatively, make a tea as you'll typically with water, adding milk to dilute) and leave this to chill inside the fridge until you intend to use it.

For the recipe, You can decide to use Bantha milk AKA 'Blue Milk', as your base. This drink is a nice butterfly pea flower, and lavender coconut milk (inspired by the Star

Wars blue milk) along with the mix of flavors using the pearls is certainly delicious.

TheActions:

Supply the warm sugary boba into a cup or glass (use glass for an excellent visual effect) and roll the cup/glass to coat the walls with melted sugar.

- Tapioca Pearls
- Tapioca Pearls and sugar
- Bantha Milk Tapioca

Then put ice (optional) as well as your liquid - the cold brew tea/iced tea, flavored milk, juice, or smoothie.
You can even top it with some whipped cream and serve.

Ways to Create Bubble Tea

Content June, everyone! It's officially summer, which for me means bubble tea season. Whom am I kidding? It's a bubble tea season for me throughout the year. However, my consumption of the stuff probably triples through the summer. Some would state it is a little bit of an addiction, but I articulate it is a means of life. Long story short, I am super excited to talk about this recipe along with you today!

Quench your thirst with refreshing, healthy, homemade bubble tea. Have a look at three easy, guilt-free recipes today!

And for a lot more excitement, I am sharing three various ways to create bubble tea:

- Simple Bubble Tea
- Milk Bubble Tea
- Fruity Bubble Tea

So why help to make bubble tea in the home? For starters, it is a breeze. Second, it is healthy! Specifically for the fruity milk teas. Consider, actual fruit vs. fruit syrup. It's instead a no brainer. Third, it is much cheaper than paying you to mix a few ingredients definitely. And finally, the comfort of whipping up a batch of the from your home means you can relax in the house and soak in sunlight on your balcony without stepping a foot out of your property or into your vehicle.

Quench your thirst with refreshing, healthy, homemade bubble tea. Have a look at three easy, guilt-free recipes today!

Tapioca Pearls

You'll need tapioca pearls because of this recipe because obviously, you can't make bubble tea with no "bubbles." Tapioca pearls can be bought online or at any nearby Asian supermarket.

You'll also need wide straws to have the ability to accommodate the pearls. These can also exist purchased online or at your neighbourhood Asian supermarket.

Ingredients
Pearls:

- ✓ 1 cup dried (boba) tapioca pearls
- ✓ 1 and 1/2 tablespoons honey.

Basic Bubble Tea:

- ✓ 1 cup tea or flavored iced tea
- ✓ lemon slice
- ✓ 3-4 ice cubes.

Milk Bubble Tea:

- ✓ 1 cup unsweetened black tea (or green tea extract)
- ✓ 1/2 cup milk or almond milk

✓ 3-4 ice cubes

Fruity Bubble Tea:

✓ 1 cup fruit of your decision (We used strawberry)

✓ 1 cup milk or almond milk

✓ 1 tablespoon honey

✓ 1 cup ice

Directions

In a big saucepan, bring 8 cups of water to some boil over high temperature. Bring the pearls and stir gently until linked with emotions. Float to the very best.

Turn the heat right down to medium and cook for 40 minutes, stirring occasionally.

Remove from heat, cover, and let sit for another 20 minutes.

Drain pearls and transfer to a little bowl. Mix in the honey and thoroughly coat—Reserve for five minutes.

Separate the pearls into three tall glasses.

Create the pursuing bubble teas:

Ordinary Bubble Tea: Add tea (or iced tea), ice, and lemon slice.

Milk Bubble Tea: Add tea, milk, and ice.

Fruity Bubble Tea: Blend fruit, milk, honey, and ice inside a blender until smooth. Pour into glass.

Put in a wide straw, and revel in!

NOTES

Tapioca pearls are best if used within a couple of hours of cooking. They'll slowly harden the longer they sit.

Taiwanese Bubble Tea

For 2 servings

Black Tea

- ✓ 2 cups water (480 g)
- ✓ 6 black tea bags

Tapioca Pearls and Brown Sugar Syrup

- ✓ ½ cup medium black tapioca pearls (50 g)
- ✓ 2 cups brown sugar (440 g)
- ✓ 1 cup of warm water (240 mL)

Ingredients

- ✓ ½ cup tapioca pearls (50 g), cooked

- ✓ ½ cup ice (30 g)
- ✓ brown sugar syrup, to taste
- ✓ 1 cup black tea (240 mL), chilled
- ✓ ¼ cup half & half (60 mL)

SPECIAL EQUIPMENT

- ✓ 2 wide-opening straws

Preparation

- ✓ In a medium pot over high temperature, combine water and tea bags. Bring to a boil, then take away the pan from heat and allow tea cool to room temperature.
- ✓ Bring a medium pot of water to boil over high temperature. Once the water is boiling, add the tapioca pearls and boil until softened, about 20 minutes.
- ✓ Drain the pearls via a filter.
- ✓ Place the filter using the pearls more than a medium bowl. Add the brown sugar to the filter and pour the warm water over.
- ✓ Stir to dissolve the brown sugar. Soak the pearls in brown sugar syrup for thirty minutes, then store the

bubbles and syrup separately until prepared to serve.

<u>Assemble the tea:</u> Split the pearls and ice between 2 glasses, then add the brown sugar syrup, tea, and half and half.

Stir having a wide-opening straw, then serve.

Enjoy!

Homemade Bubble Tea Recipes

The majority of us are most likely to be at the sunny beach at this time, but also for those stuck in the office think about changing their program a bit so that it is going to be easier to feel the long working summer days. What we're proposing would be to spice things up within the tea-drinking department with the best bubble tea.

Get this fun drink to be a part of your daily habits. Using its main ingredient being tapioca pearls, this jazzy beverage will come in pastel colors like pink, green or yellow and will undoubtedly cause you to feel like on Christmas already. Just how about rendering it at home?

We've collected five bubble tea recipes for you to try in the home, but to begin with, let's observe how to get ready for the lead ingredient.

How to cook Tapioca Pearls
Ingredients:

- ✓ six to eight 8 cups water (the ration is the very least 7:1 water to tapioca pearls)
- ✓ 1 cup tapioca pearls

Preparation:

In a big pot (Make sure the pot is big enough so boiling tapioca water won't spill over) over high temperature, add water and bring to a boil.

Slowly stir inside the tapioca pearls so that they usually do not stick together (after 1 minute, the tapioca pearls should float). Reduce heat to medium and let boil, covered, for about quarter-hour; turn the heat off and allow tapioca pearls sit, covered, for yet another a quarter-hour. After quarter-hour, remove from heat, rinse the tapioca pearls in cool water, and drain.

Mango bubble tea

This flavor will transport you with an exotic island using the first sip.

Ingredients:

- ✓ 2 green tea extract bags
- ✓ 250ml boiling water
- ✓ 1-2 tbsp honey
- ✓ 1½ litres water
- ✓ 75g large tapioca pearls
- ✓ Flesh from 1 ripe mango
- ✓ Juice of 2 oranges
- ✓ 200ml coconut milk

Preparation:

Place the teabags within the boiling water for five minutes. Take away the bags before stirring inside the honey. Reserve to cool and refrigerate until chilled.

Bring 1½ litres of water for the boil. Add the tapioca and decrease the heat into a simmer for 50 minutes, before tapioca is usually tender. Drain and rinse under cool water. Utilizing a stick blender or liquidizer, blend the mango flesh using the orange juice and coconut milk. Mix the mango liquid using the tea water as well as the tapioca. Serve in tall glasses with straws.

Jasmine pleasure bubble tea

Something is relaxing about jasmine tea, and however, in this case, it'll come out of its safe place.

Ingredients:

- ✓ 1 cup of sugar
- ✓ 1 cup large tapioca pearls
- ✓ 6 jasmine tea (or jasmine and green tea extract) bags
- ✓ 1/2 cup sweetened condensed milk

Preparation:

Put 6 jasmine tea bags right into a heat-proof container and pour over 4 cups boiling water. Let steep 20 minutes. Take away the bags and discard them. Allow tea cool, and refrigerate. If you are prepared to serve, put 1/2 cup tapioca pearls into the bottom of a big glass.

Within a pitcher, combine the tea and sweetened condensed milk and stir until blended. Pour on the pearls and serve with a supplementary large straw

English breakfast bubble tea

If you're a fan of black tea, start your mornings with this fine, bubbly recipe.

Ingredients:

- ✓ 2 English breakfast tea bags
- ✓ 2 tablespoons caster sugar
- ✓ 1 cup boiling water
- ✓ 1/4 cup tapioca
- ✓ 1 cup milk
- ✓ 1 cup ice

Preparation:

- ✓ Place tea bags, sugar, and boiling water within a heatproof jug. Stir to dissolve sugar. Reserve for five minutes for flavors to build up. Remove tea bags. Refrigerate mixture until cool.
- ✓ Bring 1.5 litres cool water towards the boil inside a saucepan over high temperature. Supply tapioca. Reduce heat to medium-low. Cook, occasionally stirring, for 45 to 50 minutes or until tapioca is

merely tender and almost clear. Drain. Rinse under cool water. Transfer to a big jug.

✓ Put tea mixture and milk to tapioca. Stir softly to combine. Separate ice between chilled glasses. Top with tapioca mixture. Serve.

Melon bubble tea

Perhaps you have ever wondered what summer taste like? You'll know after trying this recipe.

Ingredients:

✓ 2 cups prepared brewed green tea extract

✓ 1/3 cup sugar

✓ 4 cups of water

✓ 1/2 cup pearl tapioca (Raw, black or pastel-colored)

✓ 4 cups honeydews or 4 cups cantaloupes or 4 cups watermelon, chunks

✓ 4 cups ice

✓ 2 cups orange juice

✓ 1/2 cup coconut milk

Preparation:

Combine green tea extract with sugar and reserve. Drain and rinse under cool water. Combine in a medium bowl with sweetened tea. Refrigerate until needed. Blending in 2 batches, combine melon, ice, orange juice, and coconut milk in blender or food processor. Process until smooth. Place about 1/4 cup tapioca mixture in bottom of a large glass. Fill with melon mixture. Serve with straws if desired.

Matcha bubble tea

The list wouldn't be complete without a matching recipe.

Ingredients:

- ✓ 50g large tapioca pearls
- ✓ 750ml milk
- ✓ 2 tablespoons matcha powder
- ✓ 80g sugar

Preparation

Cook the tapioca pearls in a big pot of boiling water. The cooking period will vary with regards to the brand. There's an instant cook variety in Asian shops that I used here.

After the pearls are cooked, drain well and keep them in a bowl.

Bring the milk for the boil and add sugar and matcha powder. Stir until everything is dissolved. Taste to find out if you're happy with the amount of sweetness. Cool the milk mixture in the refrigerator. Serve cold within a glass using the cooked tapioca pearls and crushed ice if preferred.

Get hold of a straw and a tall glass and revel in the bubbly drink. You may make your recipe by replacing the tea together with your favorite blend. You're surely never likely to get fed up with it. The miracles of water!

Chapter 6

Health Importance of Bubble Tea

How to Determine the Best Bubble Tea

You can customize bubble tea; however, you would like. Bubble tea shop menus could be pretty complicated, but they're typically organized with grids and sub-sections to help significantly guide your ordering procedure. All you need to remember may be the classic formula: tea, milk, boba, and flavour. Don't need to select your own? Opt for a premade one. A whole lot of tea shops have their combos to consider the strain out of choosing between your hundreds of choices.

Start Using The Tea

The tea could be green, black, chai, Thai, oolong, or Pu-erh. Tea is filled with antioxidants, and green tea extract, in particular, offers one of the better waist-whittling compounds available: EGCG, an antioxidant within green tea extract, boosts your metabolism, which escalates the release of fat from stomach fat cells and increases the liver's fat-burning capacity. And green tea extract isn't the only real magic elixir. Research shows us that this antioxidant within all teas (as they're all created from the same plant) might help increase your metabolism, melt stomach fat, fight off diseases as well as reduce your threat of heart stroke and coronary disease. The drink has such a solid capability to revolutionize your waist that test panelists lost as much as 10 pounds with this best-selling plan, The 7-Day Flat-Belly Tea Cleanse!

Dairy Milk or Non-Dairy

A crucial area of the bubble tea is milk. The milk could be dairy or non-dairy, numerous shops offering soy, coconut, almond, or dairy milk and lactose-free creamers. Be certain you are getting fresh dairy food as opposed to the canned, condensed milk variety. These condensed milk are cut with plenty of prepared ingredients, and artificially sweetened-they could be around 45 percent sugar!-to make sure they are quite heavy and overpowering.

Pick Your Flavor

That is why you observe bubble teas in that broad selection of bright colours. But, it is also where ordering will get complicated. Bubble teas have flavored (and non-flavored) syrups that control the taste and colour of your tea, along with just how much sweetness is added. From *cookie dough, salted caramel, rose, cherry, coconut, melon, strawberry, taro, chocolate, sesame, almond, lavender, peppermint, as well as coffee may be used to flavor the drink.* If you like the right stuff, add *fruit, bits of mango, strawberry, apple, orange, blueberry, peach, pineapple or pomegranate seeds among countless others.* Fruity flavors pair well with plain teas, and neutral flavors like chocolate, caramel, and coconut pair well with milk teas.

Tapioca Balls or Jelly

Like the competition among tea shops upon the invention of bubble tea, tea shops remain trying methods to differentiate themselves from new establishments by supplying a wide range of toppings. Boba isn't the thing put into bubble teas now. You can even obtain popping boba, jelly, and pudding. For pudding teas, the barista can blend the complete pudding into the drink rather than adding a flavoring. Be cautious about your mixtures, though. The tartness from the fruit jelly and popping boba might not always pair well using the creaminess in the milk.

You Determine How Much Sugar You Want

With each one of these add-ons, the sugar content can genuinely add up. It's within the pearls, the milk, the syrups, as well as the fruit. Luckily, most tea shops offer clearly-defined options for degrees of sugar, such as none, 25 percent, 50 percent, 75 percent, or completely. Be careful, unless you specify sweetness, the typical or "normal" for the most part shops is complete. To be sure you're obtaining precisely the correct amount, some stores make use of a refractometer. This instrument measures the sugar content by calculating the change in wavelengths with the drink due to the current presence of sugar molecules.

Your Drink Could be Shaken or Blended

Classic iced bubble teas are chilled by shaking them with ice inside a cocktail mixer or with a machine. Just like a thicker drink, you can even get the bubble tea blended with ice, so that it has an even more smoothie-like consistency, or try making a smoothie for weight loss in the home.

Do You Prefer Your Tea with Sugar?

Even though the essential ingredients of the tea beverage could be healthy independently, when they're drowned in an excessive amount of sweetener, artificial flavor, or processed ingredients, all of the nutrition is dropped.

Once we saw earlier, the pearls are mostly made up of carbs-and not the nutritious, fiber-rich kinds within whole grains-and sugar-in the pearls themselves and in the cooking method. Also, the boba contains empty calories, not forgetting what will come in the excess syrups, and bubble tea can simply top 300 to 400 calories.

- We can not stress it enough: Watch your sweetness levels. Consuming way too many added sugars-especially those within drinks-has been associated with an increased threat of type 2 diabetes, obesity, cardiovascular disease, as well as cancer.

According to a report inside the American Journal of Clinical Nutrition, because energy from fluids offers been shown to become less satisfying than calories from food, we tend to drink much more before we feel satisfied, and you're drinking some pretty sugary things. Try choosing bubble teas with real fruit instead of artificial sweeteners and unsweetened milk. Sugars that occur naturally in foods like fruit and milk aren't the types of added sugar you should be worried about because they're combined with vitamins, minerals, and fiber.

Explanations on why Milk Tea is Wonderful for Your Health

Did you know bubble tea, which is currently popularly called pearl milk tea, continues to be existing because of the 80's decade, and it started in Taiwan around that point? When you have been drinking milk tea because it's the trend nowadays and you intend to opt for it, reconsider. There are several health advantages of milk tea that may bring you, and we are emphasizing here, 10 of these.

As mentioned, there are numerous health advantages of tea. Adding milk to the beverage helps it be not just even more flavorful but advantageous, as well. The free radicals and antioxidants in tea are what make sure they are worthier to drink. Here are the ten various other explanations why you ought to drink milk tea:

Provides strength for your body

Apart from the compounds above, milk includes a large number of different components, rendering it ideal for health. First, milk makes your body stronger. Specifically, its calcium content makes the bone stronger that can be done your day to day activities efficiently, a great way to obtain energy.

Undoubtedly, one glass of milk produces energy for your body to function well. The carb content material, as well as the different elements of milk, has also made your body stronger, leading to too much vigor. Therefore, considerably more things can be carried out once you drink milk.

Fairer and softer skin

For a long time now, just about everyone has believed that milk makes the skin we have appearance bright and good. Therefore, great medical things about milk aren't just for the body, but the skin we have, as well.

Reduces stress

Generally, our stress originates from lots of things. Whenever you drink milk tea, you'll be less stressed in virtually any given situation as milk itself, decreases tension.

Refreshes your body

Milk tea has caffeine, too, which refreshes your body. Functions as an anti-inflammatory
Milk tea comes with an anti-inflammatory agent functioning as an antioxidant in tea.

Effective for weight loss

Milk tea may also function as a realtor for both fattening and weight reduction. If you wish to gain weight, system.drawing.bitmap compound of milk in milk tea might help. And, if you want to slim down, milk tea works too, being a dietary agent from the polyphenol and caffeine. They are compounds in milk tea that help shed weight.

Stress-resistant

Apart from reducing stress, milk tea functions as an antioxidant too, which resists pressure.

Mood enhancer

With this milk tea, you will also be drinking black tea. The black tea, alternatively, includes a component called I-theanine, which boosts or enhances an excellent mood.

Creates a consistently positive feeling

Milk tea generally includes an excellent taste, and drinking a beverage having a flavour you prefer offers you that positive feeling, right? Also, just thinking about all the health advantages milk tea brings has already been reason enough to feel great while drinking it.

Best for the heart

If you drink much more than 3 cups of tea alone, it could cut the threat of heart problems. Based on the Daily Telegraph, tea alone can fortify the bone. The chance could even be reduced when the tea is blended with tea as milk has a great many other health benefits, which you can match the tea health advantages.

What makes the Tea Healthy

This content milk tea generally has, exactly why lots of people nonetheless consider it a wholesome drink. Three of the very most prevalent compounds specifically get this to popular drink an advantageous beverage:

- **Carbohydrate:** Regularly drinking one glass of milk provides energy for the body due to the carbs it includes. Don't most of us need carbohydrates to improve our strength and efficiently focus on all our actions for your day?

- **Mineral:** That is probably one of the most vital components within Milk Tea, as well, that your body needs. Minerals possess various functions in the torso.

- **Calcium:** This is the 1st compound milk has. It is one of the elements your body needs, specifically for an increasing child. The calcium in milk functions well for the bone, and the great thing about it is the fact that actually, adults can consume milk filled up with calcium.

Disadvantages of Excessive Consumption

Milk tea is a superb alternative as well as a replacement to soda if you're a regular drinker of the beverage. But despite its health advantages, it is, however, necessary to know your limitations with regards to how often and just how much you ought to drink. Health research discovered that an excessive amount of consumption of milk tea could result in specific health issues like diabetes, for just one. Below are a number of the adverse effects you may encounter;

Anxiety

While several teas like chamomile and green tea extract are well-known for their soothing houses, at times, you will find unwanted effects too, mainly if you might have excessively consumed them like anxiety, for just one. Even though tea activates the mind cells for calming down, if you drink an excessive amount of it, it could result in a brain imbalance, which, subsequently, results in anxiety.

Insomnia

Overloading with caffeine, which milk tea provides, can lead to sleep disorders such as insomnia. As with coffee, tea, mainly black tea, an ingredient for brewing milk tea is caffeine-filled. And, whenever your body is filled up with this component, especially in the afternoon, it could bring about insomnia.

Oily skin and pimples

Probably one of the most apparent unwanted effects of milk tea may be the appearance of pimples, specifically on your face if you drink sufficiently, milk tea assists with detoxifying the body. However, excessive drinking can generate an excessive amount of heat and create a body chemicals imbalance, which may bring about pimples outbreak.

Constipation

The caffeine tea contains a kind of a chemical referred to as theophylline. If you excessively drink the milk tea, the said chemical can result in extreme constipation because of the dryness and dehydration it brings to the body.

May bring about Type 2 Diabetes

Here's one bad news about drinking an excessive amount of milk tea fans. If you don't scale back on this guilty pleasure, you might be susceptible to acquiring Type 2 diabetes. Health experts recommend this milk tea every week, which is a hefty serving, and that's it.

Chapter 7

How Best is Bubble Tea to Health?

Bubble tea may have a poor reputation because of cases where it poisoned some users. However, if you pick the proper ingredients and prevent adding excess sugar, bubble tea could be healthy. In the typical tea shop, bubble tea usually includes condensed milk and sugar, which escalates the calories on the beverage, thus rendering it into the unhealthy range. However, you can find healthy alternatives to get ready for this drink, mainly if you are rendering it at home. Which means it's possible to have indeed an utterly healthy version of bubble tea, which presents you with a range of substantial health advantages;

Strengthens The Disease Fighting Capability

Green tea is among the most popular flavours of bubble tea, and it's recognized to contain numerous antioxidants like catechins that assist the disease fighting capability through the prevention of oxidative stress. Moreover, adding fruit to the drink, like strawberry or mango, also offers you a considerable dose of vitamin C, which further improves the immune system.

Energy Boost

The caffeine and sugar within green, black, or white tea get this to famous Taiwanese beverage loaded with energy. When you do not need to overdo this drink, a wholesome version with less sugar can boost your metabolism. The caffeine and sugar within green, black, or white tea get this to famous Taiwanese beverage loaded with energy. When you do not desire to overdo this drink, a wholesome version with less sugar can boost your metabolism.

Heart Health

A sugar-rich and high-calorie diet aren't always perfect for your cardiovascular well-being, but if you make a wholesome version of bubble tea, the anti-inflammatory compounds and antioxidants within the drink can fortify the blood vessel walls and stop the arteries from forming plaque.

Please take into account that these benefits are widely negated, invest an average, calorie, and sugar-rich bubble tea. The ultimate way to take pleasure in the health benefits is usually by preparing your own healthier version from the beverage in the home.

Bubble tea shops are showing up everywhere in malls, on corners, and somewhere else, thirsty teens tend to gather. Bubble tea, also known as pearl milk tea or boba tea, started in Taiwan and has turned into worldwide sipping - and chewing - phenomenon.

But what's bubble tea anyway?

Have a cup, plop in a small number of round, gelatinous pearls of tapioca, top it with brewed black or green tea extract, mix in a few milk, sugar, flavoring, and ice. Then shake everything up, and you have yourself a bubble tea.

Strangely enough, the "bubbles" in bubble tea aren't those starchy tapioca pearls, which act like the tiny black spheres of cassava you'd find in tapioca pudding. No, the "bubble" originates from what sort of drink bubbles up when it's shaken. The 1st bubble tea didn't contain tapioca pearls whatsoever.

Due to the shaking required, most bubble tea shops seal their plastic cups with cellophane and present customers a straw to poke through the very best. How big is the straw can vary greatly, with regards to the size of the tapioca pearls: smaller pearls, thinner straw. To sip the more prevalent 6-millimeter pearls, you may need a fatter straw. Adventurous sippers then pop their straw through the most notable and revel in or not. Some liken the conscious connection with drinking bubble tea with tapioca pearls to drinking a smoothie filled with gummy bears. The tapioca pearls lend texture to drinking that some cannot get accustomed to (it is odd to need to chew a beverage).

If that sounds appealing to you, it is a matter of personal taste. Some individuals create a full-blown bubble tea habit, downing the drinks every single day, especially during warmer seasons. And with an array of flavors, i.e., red bean, avocado, taro root, coconut, guava, ginger, jack fruit, watermelon, mango, lemon, lychee, mocha, sesame, strawberry, the list could continue and on - you could attempt a fresh bubble tea every day.

But would that be such an excellent idea?

To obtain a better notion of bubble tea's nutritional profile, we have to go through the main ingredients. The bottom of bubble tea usually is black or green tea extract. Tea is a low-fat, low-calorie beverage rich with cell-supporting antioxidants. *Though tea generally contains less caffeine than coffee, it affects everyone differently. Look out for restlessness, irritability, and disturbed sleep.* To include a hint of fruity flavour, bubble tea establishments will sometimes add a purée of fruit (excellent!). Unfortunately, many shops go the cost-effective route, using fruit syrups, which may be saturated in sugar and all of the fat and calories that are included.

Milk products put in a creamy thickness to bubble tea; however, they also put fat and calories, and so are a pain for those who have lactose intolerance. Pure bubble tea has 160 calories. Swirl milk in, and it rises to 230 calories.

Ask in case a shop can forgo condensed milk towards soy milk, low-fat milk, or non-dairy creamers.

And sorry to burst your bubble, but tapioca pearls place boba tea's calorie count firmly in the "Yikes!" category. Once you plop pearls into the milky tea, you are looking at over 300 calories - and much more sugar! Some estimates declare that just one single ounce of tapioca pearls contains 100 calories. Due to the fact recipes demand 2-3 ounces of pearls per cup of tea, you're sucking back some significant calories.

Still around the bubble about bubble tea? Like other delightfully decadent drinkables - think ice-whipped lattes and mega-sized smoothies - bubble tea is more of meals or perhaps a dessert when compared to a beverage to quench your thirst. Consider bubble tea one particular indulgence to savour occasionally, when you wish something cool, creamy, fruity - and slightly bit chewy!

How Healthy is Bubble Tea to Human?

Bubble tea could be healthy if you choose the best ingredients and prevent adding excess sugar to the beverage. Within an average tea store, it'll often include condensed milk and extra sugar, boosting the entire calorie count in the drink and pushing it into the unhealthy realm. However, you will find healthier methods to prepare this beverage, especially if you are rendering it for yourself in the home.

Benefits

This exotic tea offers benefits that are the following:

Boosts Energy

Due to the sugar in bubble tea, as well as the caffeine that's within black, white, or green tea extract, this popular Taiwanese drink can offer a significant boost in energy. When you don't wish to overdo this beverage, given its high calorie and sugar count number, a wholesome version with less sugar could still give a kickstart for your metabolism.

Strengthens Disease Fighting Capability

Green tea, probably one of the most popular flavours of bubble tea, contains an array of antioxidants such as catechins and polyphenols, which can enhance the disease fighting capability by preventing oxidative stress. Furthermore, if you choose fruits within your tea such as mango, strawberry or kiwi, you'll also get yourself a dose of vitamin C inside your tea, meaning a lot more of the boost for the disease fighting capability.

Prevents Free Radical Damage

The polyphenols and epigallocatechin within green bubble tea can have impressive effects within the free radicals going swimming the body. These free radicals could cause mutation and result in chronic diseases and cancer, so adding green tea extract to your daily diet is always a great choice. However, further research and studies are needed. A sugar-rich diet isn't always best for your cardiovascular health, however in the situation of boba tea, if you make a healthy version, the antioxidants and anti-inflammatory compounds within the tea can help maintain healthy body and heart.

Note: These health advantages are largely negated whenever you drink a standard, sugar-rich, and calorie-heavy bubble tea. Creating your own healthier versions in the home is usually highly suggested if you wish to enjoy these effects.

Chapter 8

Bubble Tea Tips

Bubble tea was invented in Taiwan, as well as the "bubble" a part of its brand identifies the foam you get from shaking it.

Bubble tea is a drink that is around for a lot more than 30 years," Phan says. It had been invented in Taiwan within the 1980s, and it's traditionally a milk tea. It's freshly brewed tea with milk and sugar, which has been shaken with ice inside a cocktail shaker - that is where the word 'bubble tea' originates. Shaking the tea gives it a bubble foam together with the drink, and that's its namesake!

Why Is Bubble Tea Unique?

Toppings are in the bottom from the drink, and also you drink it with an enormous straw, so bubble tea is similar to a combination between food and a glass or two; it's just like a drink snack.

Lots of people whenever they start to see the toppings move 'Oh', that's bubble tea!' therefore i believe that's its defining factor.

The Original & Most Common "Topping" is

Tapioca Pearls.

Tapioca pearls will be the black balls you observe at the bottom of the drink. Tapioca is a starch that originates from the cassava root. It's rolled within a shot, and we cook it fresh here. It must be boiled and prepared, and it could be flavored with almost any sugar or syrup you want. We flavour it with brown sugar here.

It's slightly sweet and slightly chewy and includes a very addictive texture. It's a thing that people call 'Kue' texture - we have a whole lot of foods with this sort of chewy texture, like mochi.

You can use jellies and popping boba as toppings.

The jellies used are called 'nata de coco,' and so are from your Philippines. They're created from coconut water. They ferment the normal coconut water, which allows it to jellify; however, they don't bring gelatin or anything like this - it's vegan and gluten-free, then flavour it with the addition of juices or fruit syrups to it.

We import our popping boba; we don't make sure they are. They're filled up with juice or fruit puree, and they've made through an activity called spherification, that you may have seen at some fancy restaurants. It's created by dropping acidic juice into an algae cellulose calcium solution that naturally forms a skin around it.

You can judge how sound a bubble tea shop is by the tapioca pearls.

For me, the mark of an excellent bubble tea place may be the tapioca pearls. Everyone includes a personal preference, but I love them to exist quite chewy but soft, and I love to have the ability to chew each pearl five or six times. When you have to eat the pearl 20 times, then it's too much and too chewy. If it reduces in the mouth area after two bites, then it's likely a little stale or continues to be overcooked.

We help to make our pearls fresh every two hours. The grade of the pearl is a good gauge of if the bubble tea shop is making things fresh and if they care about the grade of their drink.

The toppings could be a choking hazard, so don't give bubble tea to small children, and be cautious!

Choking is something first-timers may be at risk of, as they're not used to bubble tea. Especially in the united kingdom, individuals are not used to presenting their tea with bits in it! Just drinking it slowly and trying to only have 3 to 4 bits of topping in the mouth area at onetime help. Don't go prematurely.

You may swallow the entire bubble if you want, but it sort of defeats the reason because they're chewy. Also, don't give bubble tea to children below four years of age, as the bubble is a choking hazard to them."

If you'd like, you can order bubble tea without toppings.

Classic milk tea may be the original bubble tea flavour, and it's nonetheless typically the most popular.

Plenty of places just call it classic milk tea; that's usually the most popular flavour. It's black tea with milk powder and sugar.

We don't call our classic milk tea, though, because we avoid milk powder - we call our version Hong-Kong-style milk tea. It's classic milk tea made out of evaporated milk instead of powder. We make it by brewing strong black tea, which we then strain and cool by pulling the liquid.

We then add evaporated milk directly to make it spare creamy and further thick. It's our top-selling flavor.

You may make classic bubble tea in the home.

If you wish to make a regular bubble tea in the home, select a black tea something substantial as an Assam and brew it inside a teapot. Make sure to brew it for longer than you usually would. Then mix this using the large amount of the very best quality milk you'll find. Bring the sugar to your liking bubble tea has a whole lot of sugar traditionally, but folks are adding less sugar nowadays. Contribute ice, shake it within a cocktail shaker, and you have bubble tea!

The hard part is the tapioca pearls. It's hard to create that in the home. You get the pearls dry (we import ours from Taiwan; nevertheless, you will get them in Chinatown), then cook these to encourage them to the chewy texture. I'd say it often takes about 40 minutes of preparation and cooking period, which is a lot of periods spent trying to create one drink in the home. I'd just recommend making bubble tea yourself if you're carrying it out for any big party."

Nowadays, there are loads of different varieties of bubble tea; milk tea, ice tea, fruity milk, mousse tea, as well as coconut water tea!

Bubble tea has evolved a whole lot during the last 30 years and be a vast category. Milk tea is your most traditional kind of bubble tea. That is just various kinds of tea with milk; it could be rooibos, jasmine, genmaicha, Assam. It's merely tea with milk and toppings added. I don't want to stereotype, but this is precisely what customers from Parts of Asia choose to drink because that's what we should suppose bubble tea is: milk tea with tapioca.

Then you possess ice tea, which is commonly more popular in the united kingdom. Ice tea could be any tea, but with different fruit flavours added, instead of milk. Here, we add fruit nectars that are fruit juices that have been converted to nectars for all of us.

You can even get fruity milk teas that are like milkshakes, but less bulky once we don't need use ice cream. It's milk or milk powder with fruit nectar or syrup put into flavour it.

There are always new types of bubble tea being invented, though. For example, we recently invented the coconut water bubble tea. It's just pure coconut water having a little bit of fruit nectar added in if you'd like, you'll be able to contribute toppings to it."

If you'd like something different, order mousse bubble tea.

Mousse bubble tea is relatively unique. It's various kinds of pure tea in the bottom with a little bit of sugar put into sweetening it. Then we top it having a whipped savoury mousse. It's definitely for those who tend to be more adventurous. It offers you a two-layer drink, which people tend only to mix immediately, and produces a vibrant, creamy sweet and savoury tea. We make it with a little secret ingredient and whipping cream."

If you wish to look like an expert, there is a trick to putting your straw within your drink.

If you simply bang your straw with the plastic, it'll produce the tea leak from the opening. Instead, put your thumb at the top with the straw to create an airtight seal, then confidently stab along. That's the proper way to put your straw in. When someone does, you could tell they're an expert."

Taro milk tea can be an unexpectedly good flavour.

Anyone who knows bubble tea knows taro is impressive. It's a cult favourite among bubble tea lovers. It's made out of taro root and yams, but a sensible way to describe the taste of it is cookies and cream. It tastes like cookies and cream."

If you are a first-timer, either order the classic milk tea or if you wish to fun it very safe, and ice tea.

If you're trying bubble tea for the very first time, and you intend to try authentic bubble tea, I'd say choose the classic milk bubble tea with tapioca pearls. That's probably the most traditional definition of just what a bubble tea can be in my own eyes.

But if you wish to take it up safe, everyone likes an iced peach tea or passion fruit tea, especially on the hot day.

It's so refreshing - we've never really had anyone try not to go 'wow.'

Bubble tea is gluten-free and may become as healthy while you want to buy to be.

The overall perception of bubble tea is the fact that it's not so healthy, as it's traditionally made out of artificial ingredients, the tea isn't fresh, and there's a whole lot of sugar used.

We're trying to improve that at this moment causing healthier, even more, natural bubble tea. We do this by producing the tea fresh. Bubble tea is traditionally created by brewing plenty of tea each day and keeping it during the day. Tea is abundant with antioxidants, but antioxidants deteriorate, so you're not likely to get as many health advantages from tea that hasn't been brewed fresh.

Other areas also use powdered creamer, which includes plenty of artificial chemicals in it, plus vegetable oils and trans fats. Here we use organic fresh milk. We also provide you with the substitute for customising your sugar too, you could have full sugar, half sugar, or no sugar, or we can swap the sugar for honey. We also offer organic chia seeds like a topping, but all our toppings are gluten-free too. It could be as healthy when you want it to become.

Zero-calorie bubble tea does exist; however, the healthiest bubble tea is a matcha bubble tea.

Here we can produce a close-to-zero-calorie drink: pure ice tea with zero sugar and chia seeds.

But if you need a nutritious instead of zero-calorie drink though, I'd get a *matcha bubble tea*. I'd say that's the healthiest bubble tea. Matcha has plenty of health advantages; it's like green tea extract x 10. Have that without sugar and either fresh organic milk or, if you'd like no dairy, order it with almond milk, then top it with organic chia seeds."

Bubble tea over here isn't that dissimilar to bubble tea in Taiwan.

To be completely honest, I believe the bubble tea you overcome here is nearly the same as the bubble tea you enter Taiwan. Most of the brands are from Taiwan, or make use of ingredients they import from Taiwan. The only real difference is the fact Taiwanese bubble tea shops are more complex.

"I head to Taiwan often to accomplish research, plus the last period I had been there having been several brands doing fresh milk only. One brand was only doing fruit, and one brand was only making fresh tea. They're moving towards more natural and sweet bubble tea.

"They've had it for 30 to 40 years now, so they're pros at drinking it. It's like their coffee. When you go to Taipei, every street has at least one bubble tea place. They're now very alert to what goes into their bubble tea. Within the UK, folks are nonetheless not alert to what bubble tea is and what switches into it."

The bubble tea flavours that tend to confuse many people are Thai milk tea, winter melon, and genmaicha.

Thai milk tea is quite famous and can be made out of evaporated milk. It's traditionally an adorable drink, but we get ours less sweet. It's orange because in Thailand they put in a little bit of food colouring to it. If you discover an orange drink, you understand it's Thai tea. It tastes sort of *vanilla-y*.

Winter melon may be the most confusing drink we've, as a whole lot of customers can be found in and think they're obtaining watermelon flavour if they order it. It's an extremely traditional Chinese melon, so when you cook it, it caramelizes, so it's an extremely smoky, caramel flavour. Contrary to watermelon!

Genamaicha is Japanese green tea extract, which is green tea extract that's been blended with the toasted grain. Some individuals call it popcorn tea, as the flavour you reach the end can be a popcorn-like toasted grain flavour.

Drink your bubble tea once you can. There is nothing like newly shaken bubble tea!

You ought to drink bubble tea once you can. Get yourself a large number of people who has delivery or take it away and drink it the very next day. Still, I believe it's always better to drink it on a single daytime you order it mainly if the drink is using fresh milk instead of powder, and if you haven't had bubble tea before, definitely come check it out! A lot of people either enjoy it or at least recognize it's a fresh experience. It's an enjoyable way to drink tea!

Chapter 9

The Taxonomy

Classic Milk Tea

Black tea is shaken with frothy milk, crushed ice, and some generous handfuls of marble-sized, caramelized tapioca pearls. There are versions with different kinds of milk and different teas; however, the classic still satisfies.

Brown Sugar

Ultra-rich brown sugar boba tea has been an explosive hit in Taiwan, made popular partly because of the chain Tiger Sugar - a milk-heavy boba drink doused using a generous shot of cloyingly sweet brown sugar syrup, all swirling in a lovely gradient of cocoa-browns and teeth.

Taro Milk Tea

Taro bubble tea started in Taiwan inside the 1980s and later swept throughout Asia along with the West. Notable because of its colour, which runs from purple-tinged brown to nearly lilac, and its coconut-like flavour, taro (a root vegetable similar to a sweet potato) is pureed and put into boba milk tea, where it acts being a thickener and flavoring.

Fruit-Filled

If milk isn't in your cup of tea, you will find fresh fruit-based boba drinks that have precisely the same addictive textures. Popular flavors include mango, lychee, winter melon, lemon, as well as tomato, plus they arrive bobbing with boba pearls but also other things, like aiyu jelly (made out of the seeds of an area selection of creeping fig), watermelon cubes, and crunchy passionfruit seeds.

Fully Loaded

Add-ins own long since expanded beyond tapioca balls, and today include choices like grass jelly, aloe vera, almond jelly, custardy egg pudding, adzuki beans, panna cotta, chia seeds, sweet potato balls, even Oreo cookies because you will want to? The tapioca balls themselves have slowly evolved beyond the typical sugary taste, and today covers a wide spectral range of flavors, including sea salt, cheese, wood ear mushroom, quinoa, tomato, chocolate, Sichuan pepper, jujube, and barley.

Eye Candy

Fueled by Instagram, shops in Taiwan are churning out drinks made to look as effective as or much better than they taste, ideally while clutched sunlight completely with a freshly manicured hand. Scroll via a boba-focused feed to identify bright, spicy drinks with red-hot pearls and a sprinkling of chile powder, tie-dye versions made out of blue butterfly pea, and jet-black cups infused with inky (and detoxifying) charcoal. Some shops will also be turning toward alternative organic sweeteners like honey and agave nectar for the health-conscious.

Cheese Tea

A Taiwanese night market stand began combining powdered cheese and salt with whipping cream and milk to create a foamy, tangy layer at the top of the cup of cold tea. The cheese-topped drink is currently accessible in lots of elements of Asia and has found an audience Stateside as well.

Edibles, Cocktails, Skincare, etc.

Taking into consideration the amount of chewing already involved, it's no real surprise that boba pearls are starring in several culinary applications, working their way into from souffle pancakes, sandwiches, hot pot soup, pizza, creme brulee, and undoubtedly the stalwart, shaved ice.

For individuals who want their boba stiff, nowadays, there are boba cocktails made out of vodka, tequila, gin, rum, or bourbon. Bars throughout Taiwan and beyond are tinkering with these alcoholic boba concoctions, and LA even includes a boba-centric bar focused on liquor-filled spins on traditional boba flavors, and then, just do it, smear boba around your face if you'd like. Taiwan now offers lotions, facial blotting tissues, candles, as well as boba milk tea face masks (with real boba pearls inside), all boasting the signature, sticky-sweet fragrance of boba milk tea. Gimmicky, sure, but anything in the brand of beauty - and boba.

Order Just Like A Pro

Boba comes with its lingo. Whichever style you select, get the drink such as a local - fully customized. Here's a glossary:

- ✓ Quán táng (全糖) - Full sugar
- ✓ Shǎo táng (少糖) - Less sugar

- ✓ Bàn táng (半糖) - Half sugar

- ✓ Wēi táng (微糖) - Some sugar

- ✓ Zhèngcháng bīng (正常冰) - Regular ice

- ✓ Shǎo bīng (少冰) - Less ice

- ✓ Qù bīng (去冰) - No ice

- ✓ Wēn yǐn (溫飲) - Warm

- ✓ Rèyǐn (熱飲) - Hot

Methods of Ordering Boba Tea
Food

Boba tea, which can be referred to as bubble or pearl tea, is a beverage that started in Taiwan and is currently accessible in lots of countries. If you've heard friends and family raving concerning this drink and want to check it out on your own, then read on for some tips about ordering your first boba tea.

Decide if you'd like milk or no milk.

There are various kinds of bubble tea, but all are made either with milk or without it. If you're craving something fruity and refreshing, you might need to order a boba tea without milk. If you need a treat that is rich and creamy, then consider boba milk tea options. Although some fruit flavors are delicious when coupled with dairy, savoury varieties tend to be famous for milk teas.

Choose about the most flavours.

The most regularly ordered boba teas are favourites for grounds. When ordering your first bubble tea, you can benefit from selecting a flavour that's widely-liked, which can only help make sure that your 1st experience is usually a delicious one. Classic boba tea, which is manufactured with milk, black tea, tapioca pearls, and sweetener, is a superb substitute for considering. A number of the additional popular flavours include almond, honeydew, strawberry, taro, and coconut.

Do not get overwhelmed by toppings.

When ordering a bubble tea, you might be asked if you want any toppings. While their name suggests otherwise, most toppings sit in the bottom from the cup with regards to bubble tea. Your options for toppings may differ significantly between bubble tea shops; however, many common types include grass jelly, pudding, fruit, aloe vera, and coconut jellies. With regards to ordering your first boba tea, donâ□™t feel obligated to make a complicated drink. Instead, order a boba tea that sounds delicious for you.

Answers to Common Questions about Ordering Bubble Tea Drink

Are you wanting to try your initial bubble tea but look overwhelmed by the number of menu options? If so, then read on to understand the answers to commonly asked questions about ordering bubble tea.

What exactly are bubble tea toppings?

Although their name implies otherwise, bubble tea toppings will be the things that fall to underneath in the cup. Tapioca pearls that are generally known as boba will be the standard bubble tea topping, and so are what folks often think about when bubble tea involves mind. However, you will find other available choices that you will find to select from, such as fruit jellies, pudding, and popping boba.

Will there be a 'plain' bubble tea?

The closest thing to an ordinary bubble tea is classic milk tea, which may be the original bubble tea recipe. Classic milk tea is manufactured with black tea, as well as sweetener, milk, and tapioca pearls; this unique bubble tea flavour is relatively accessible and may be a fantastic choice for anybody trying bubble tea for the very first time. Not prepared to make an effort toppings within your drink? Then just order your bubble tea without toppings or boba.

Imagine if I don't want milk?

Bubble tea can be an incredibly customizable drink. Which means that you may order the flavour that you would like, but without the dairy added. Some flavors to consider for bubble tea without milk include pineapple, strawberry, watermelon, passion fruit, and green apple.

Our fruit flavours much better than savoury ones?

While fruit flavours are widely loved with regards to bubble tea, many people choose savoury flavours. To get your preferred bubble tea flavours, consider ordering something new every time. For savoury flavours, some popular options include coffee, avocado, red bean, taro, and coconut.

Happy TeaHouse & Café includes a wide range of delicious bubble tea flavors for you to choose from and a menu that has snacks, grain dishes, and smoothies.

Does Bubble Tea Always Include Tapioca?

Traditionally, bubble tea does include tapioca, which is often known as boba. In the end, it's the pearls in the bottom with the cup that produces bubble tea so recognizable. However, you can always customize your bubble tea drink, which means that you could order it without the tapioca.

If you're not a fan of the chewy tapioca pearls that always include bubble tea, you can merely require tea with no boba and revel in a delicious beverage. However, if you nonetheless desire your drink to get something apart from tea, milk, and flavouring, then consider adding another topping. Bubble tea shops typically provide a selection of toppings you could add to your drink, such as grass jelly, coconut candies, fruit jam, popping boba, and pudding.

Which kind of Tea Is within Bubble Tea?

As the name implies, bubble tea is traditionally made utilizing a tea base. Most bubble tea shops make their bubble tea exclusively with black tea, which is recognized as red tea in Taiwan, Hong Kong, and China. Earl Grey is among the most popular types of black tea used to create boba tea.

Although black tea is by far the predominant kind of bubble tea base, some locations offer other choices. For example, green tea extract, and particularly jasmine green tea extract, may also be used. Also, many shops include matcha green tea-flavoured boba tea on the menu. Oolong tea may also be an option, as well. Finally, some tea houses provide a selection of white tea base, which may be perfect for anyone sensitive towards the flavours of black or green tea extract.

Chapter 10

Interesting Factual Statements about
Tapioca Pearls

When a lot of people consider bubble tea, the boba pearls that fill underneath with the glass are what often one thinks of. If you're a fan of boba tea, then continue reading to understand some interesting factual statements about the chewy tapioca pearls that sit in the bottom on the cup.

They are created from a root.

Tapioca pearls are produced from tapioca starch, which starch comes from a root called cassava. Cassava root, which can be referred to as manioc or yucca, is native to Brazil and grown widely through the entire Caribbean. Cassava, which is a staple food in lots of cultures, is long and tuberous having a darkish skin and a white interior.

They could be in several colours.

Many folks are acquainted with the evident and black boba varieties. Clear boba is produced from typical tapioca pearls, and black ones are often made out of brown sugar or caramel coloring. Now, some bubble tea shops offer boba in other colors as well, such as yellow, pink, and orange.

They could be filled up with different flavors.

Black and clear boba remain the hottest boba varieties in America. However, in a few countries, boba is manufactured with flavored fillings like chocolate, red bean, and mung bean. The boba themselves may also be flavored with the addition of ingredients for the tapioca pearls because they are cooked.

They cannot play your mouth.

Lots of the colorful boba available certainly are a variety called popping boba. However, although they are called boba, these bursting bubbles aren't tapioca pearls. Instead, they are produced from seaweed extract, fruit drinks, along with other ingredients. Traditional boba created from tapioca pearls, alternatively, are notably soft and chewy.

A Guide to Ordering an ideal Bubble Tea

Bubble tea is a great and delicious drink that is growing in popularity. However, you might have questions about the various options that exist when trying this sort of drink for the very first time. Read on to understand how exactly to order an ideal bubble tea.

Temperature

However, this beverage is traditionally served cold, and these iced options are what most bubble tea shops offer on the menu.

Type

The typical bubble tea drink could be categorized as either fruity or creamy. Creamy bubble teas, which are occasionally called milk teas, come with an opaque appearance, boast a creamy consistency, and so are typically made out of milk, soy milk, or almond milk. Fruity bubble tea is a tea drink that's usually flavour-rich and incredibly refreshing.

Tea

Many boba tea shops provide an extensive collection of drink combinations for customers to select from, and some enable you to pick the kind of tea that you like. In any case, you will likely have the decision between a black tea and a green tea extract beverage. Black tea options will often have the highest levels of caffeine.

Flavour

Next, its normal to take into account what flavor you would like. Generally, creamy bubble teas work best with flavors like mocha, vanilla, and coconut. In contrast, fruit flavors like peach, passionfruit, and mango are reserved for the fruity bubble teas that are created without milk. However, creamy bubble tea mixes made out of fruit flavors certainly are a favorite for many individuals and can exist delicious, as well.

Finally, you might find that we now have some additional choices for you to consider when ordering your bubble tea. Pudding, for instance, can bring considerably more texture and rich flavor for your creamy bubble teas, while jellies and popping boba are favorites for fruit-flavoured blends.

Exploring Boba Tea and its Flavors

Drink Using the wide variety of mixtures and types that exist; boba tea often means something unique to each individual. Read on to understand a bit relating to this beverage, as well as the flavors that you may see on the menu at a bubble tea house.

Milk Tea

When boba tea is manufactured with dairy or perhaps a dairy substitute, that is known as milk tea, although milk tea could be made out of or without boba. Though it depends on personal preference, many people discover that some flavors are better fitted to milk tea than others. A few examples of popular milk tea flavors include green bean, red bean, coconut, avocado, almond, coffee, matcha green tea extract, taro, Thai tea, and mocha. There are also fruit flavors that match milk, such as honeydew, papaya, pineapple, orange, strawberry, mango, and peach.

Fruit Tea

Alternatively, some fruit flavors are popular for boba tea thatâ™s made without milk, such as cherry, lychee, green apple, cantaloupe, raspberry, passion fruit, kiwi, and lemon.

Green Tea

Traditional boba tea is manufactured utilizing a base of black tea. However, there are also plenty of bubble tea flavors that have a green tea extract base, which may be suitable for anyone who's worried about caffeine content or wants to enjoy the health advantages of green tea extract. A number of the green tea extract flavor alternatives that could be over a bubble tea menu include peppermint, jasmine, and passion fruit.

Add-Ins

As though boba tea was not already customizable enough, many add-ins exist because of this popular beverage. A few examples consist of pudding, caffeine shots, extra boba, popping boba, grass jelly, mango jelly, coffee jelly, and coconut jelly. With so many choices, you'll never go out of boba tea varieties to try.

A glance at the Various Types of Boba

If you are a fan of bubble tea, then you're probably acquainted with boba. Sometimes known as the bubbles that sit at the bottom of the bubble tea drink, the bobs are produced from a kind of tapioca pearl. Today, you'll find many types of boba.

Clear Boba

Standard boba pearls are produced from the cassava root, which is a starchy tuber that's linked to the yam. Tapioca starch is manufactured out of the cassava, which carbohydrates can then be compressed into balls to create tapioca pearls. For their apparent colour, traditional bobas could be made in an array of fun, bright colors.

Black Boba

The dark coloured tapioca pearls that certainly are a popular choice for bubble tea drinks are called black bobas. They are created just as that apparent bobas are, except with the help of caramel coloring or brown sugar to provide them with their dark color.

Flavored Boba

To improve the versatility of boba pearls, some locations offer flavored varieties. Flavored bobas are typical tapioca pearls that are cooked with or coated inside a flavored syrup. The flavor possibilities for these pearls are endless; however, many familiar favourites include honey, watermelon, orange, and strawberry.

Popping Boba

To take the idea of flavored boba a little further, popping bobas were developed. This boba variety is undoubtedly filled with juice. Once you bite down on a popping boba, it bursts within your mouth, releasing the sweet juice. Popping boba will come in many flavours, with some popular ones being mango, passionfruit, banana, and pineapple.

Mini Boba

Mini bobas, as the name implies, are much smaller. Mini bobas are about 50 % how big is regular bobas, and therefore they cook faster and smaller. Some individuals could find that mini bobas are better to chew compared to the more extensive variety.

Chapter 11

FAQs About Various Kinds of Boba

If you value trying different bubble tea flavors, you then already recognize that there will vary types of tapioca pearls you can use to produce this tasty drink. However, just how much have you any idea about each kind? Continue reading to understand the answers to common questions about types of boba.

Do Clear Boba Taste Good?

Boba pearls are produced from tapioca starch, which originates from a root vegetable called cassava. When cooked, the tapioca pearls can grow to 10 millimeters in size and be translucent. The distinct boba is incredibly versatile because it could be made virtually any colour by soaking them in a variety of liquids and syrups. However, when cooked usually, clear boba has hardly any flavor.

What makes some boba black?

You might have pointed out that most bubble tea beverages natural black tapioca pearls rather than transparent. One reason behind that is their color, which sticks out at the bottom of any bubble tea drink. The next reason behind their popularity is the fact that black boba is created using brown sugar, gives them their dark colour but also a sweet flavor. The principal differences between bright and black boba are that black ones are darker in color, and cooked with brown sugar.

Can you put flavor to boba?

Both black and clear boba could be prepared in a manner that adds flavor towards the tapioca; this is done by soaking the cooked pearls within a sweetened and flavoured syrup.

What is the difference between typical boba and pearl boba?

Boba tea and pearl tea tend to be used interchangeably to spell it out bubble tea beverages. However, some individuals consider pearl tea to get bubble tea that's made out of smaller tapioca pearls, which can be about half how wide is the more significant variety.

Tips for Deciding on The Best Boba Tea Toppings

There are so many choices for boba tea flavors and toppings that choosing an excellent combination isn't always straightforward. When ordering your beverage next time you go to a boba tea home, keep the pursuing in mind with regards to choosing your toppings:

The flavor that you decide on for the bubble tea should impact the selection of toppings. For instance, if you select a fruity boba tea flavor, such as passion fruit or green apple, a creamy topping like pudding could cause a clash of flavors. Instead, try adding creamy toppings to flavors like taro, coconut, and avocado. Conversely, the tartness of popping boba or fruit jelly won't always pair well with savoury boba tea flavors. Because of this, consider reserving fruit jelly and popping boba for boba tea flavors like pineapple, strawberry, and lychee.

Flavors of Bubble Tea

While all the other ingredients form the bottom for bubble tea (tea, milk, and boba), the real flavor originates from the flavoring ingredient like a syrup or powder. Just like coffee houses could have a fall into line of syrup bottles to flavor lattes, bubble tea shops are stocked with an excellent selection of syrups and powders.

Flavored simple syrups will be the popular flavoring option because they mix easily into the cold milk tea. Some popular fruity options include:

- ✓ Honeydew
- ✓ Lychee
- ✓ Mango
- ✓ Passion Fruit
- ✓ Peach
- ✓ Plum
- ✓ Strawberry
- ✓ Avocado
- ✓ Banana
- ✓ Cantaloupe
- ✓ Coconut
- ✓ Grape
- ✓ Green Apple
- ✓ Jackfruit
- ✓ Kiwi
- ✓ Lemon

- ✓ Pineapple
- ✓ Watermelon

For any less fruity flavour, try these popular options:

- ✓ Almond
- ✓ Coffee
- ✓ Ginger
- ✓ Pudding (e.g., chocolate, custard, mango, or taro)
- ✓ Taro
- ✓ Barley
- ✓ Caramel
- ✓ Chocolate
- ✓ Lavender
- ✓ Mocha
- ✓ Rose
- ✓ Sesame
- ✓ Bubbles
- ✓ The Spruce / Cara Cormack.

Types of Bubbles as well as Other Additions

Initially, the "bubble" within the name "bubble tea" described the environment bubbles formed by shaking in the tea and milk mixtures. However, it is now utilized to refer to the "pearls" or "boba" along with other ingredients within similar drinks. These drinks routinely have what's called "QQ" in Taiwan and China.

QQ can be a chewy texture that's adored in Chinese and Taiwanese cuisines. QQ foods need not be flavorful being popular, plus they usually aren't. The most frequent types of bubbles using the sought-after QQ qualities include:

- **Tapioca Pearls:** Small, round globules of boiled tapioca starch offering an extremely chewy, almost gum-like texture and minimal flavour. They are usually purplish-black, though they can also be white or pastel in color. They may be the most popular boba (often simply called boba) and will vary in proportions.

- **Jelly:** Grass jelly is manufactured out of Chinese mesona, the chewy cubes have a lightly sweet, herbal flavor. Aloe jelly is comparable but created from the aloe plant. Other jelly flavors like coconut are occasionally offered as well.

- **Taro Balls:** Cooked and frequently purple, these sweet balls are produced from the taro plant.

- **Nice Potato Balls:** Chewy balls made using orange sweet potato.

- **<u>Tapioca noodles</u>**: Usually created from white tapioca and shaped into thin, noodle-like strands that may be slurped up through a broad bubble tea straw.

- **<u>Pudding:</u>** Thick, creamy custard puddings that may be put into your drink being a decadent treat. Dessert typically will come in different flavors, like taro or coffee.

- **<u>Popping Boba:</u>** A undertakes the typical tapioca pearls that "pop" in the mouth area for any burst of flavor. These will come in a variety of flavor options.

Additional popular topping and mix-ins include:

- **<u>Fruit:</u>** Diced fruit is usually popular in bubble tea, especially in fruit teas

- **<u>Red Bean:</u>** Sweet, creamy red beans

- **<u>Cookie Crumbs:</u>** Crumbled up Oreos or similar cookies

- **<u>Ice Cream:</u>** Some shops offer ice cream like a mix-in or topper for bubble tea

- **<u>Cheese Cream:</u>** A sweet, salty, and savoury cream made out of cheese powder.

Best Bubble Tea Flavors

Bubble tea, or boba tea, is often a Taiwanese drink that has exploded in popularity all over the world lately. It's a delicious beverage usually created from tea, milk, sugar, and of course, tapioca pearls! Occasionally numerous kinds of jellies and puddings may also be added for something spare.

With flavors that range from melon to coffee to lavender to chocolate, bubble tea will have a flavor that suits every taste. But how will you choose from a lot of flavors? Well, we've come up with a summary of what we believe will be the ten best bubble tea flavors to start your boba journey!

Classic Milk Tea/Brown Sugar

The classic is manufactured with black tea, milk powder, sugar, and undoubtedly, tapioca pearls. Its rich and creamy flavor coupled with its smooth tea flavor will send you right to your content place. For people who have a beautiful tooth, order the brown sugar version for a straight sweeter kick! If it's your first-time drinking bubble tea or you're not feeling too adventurous, this is the perfect starter tea.

Mango

For those having a fruity palate and a tropical flair, this is the bubble tea for you personally. Mango, inside our personal opinion, is most beneficial to drink in slushie form. Yes, they have bubble tea slushies! Or they can possess the consistency of shaved iced based on where you proceed. When it's a hot, summer day, what could be much better than a cold drink which allows you to drift away to your preferred beach destination?

Honeydew

Probably one of the most popular flavours worldwide, this melon drink can be amazingly refreshing inside the blazing summer heat. It's also an ideal way to combine drinking boba while also getting your nutrients! Although many places will include a lot of added sugar, it's a good idea to ask for it. If you love fruit, this is your drink to start with. Be adventurous, and find out why this is the staple flavour of so many Asian households.

Thai Tea

Thai tea is sweeping the country with it's creamy, excellent uniqueness. The orange colour originates from a special sort of tea called Ceylon tea, which is probably one of the most popular bases for iced tea on the planet. Although sadly, the intense brightness from the orange may be from assistance from food colouring (make sure to ask when ordering). In any event, this flavor brings the streets of Thailand right to the mouth area. The just thing better than Thai tea is Thai bubble tea!

Taro

This fun purple drink is manufactured out of a slightly sweet Asian root called Taro. Don't allow a unique name or colour scare you away, or you're sure to regret it. Taro is challenging to spell it out but is usually believed to have a nutty, earthy, vanilla-Esque flavour. Many people swear it tastes exactly like cookies and cream. You choose!

Strawberry

Recreate childhood memory with this fresh undertake the easy but delicious strawberry milk. Slightly tangy, but oh so sweet, strawberries are America's closest friend. Now within a lot more interesting way. Slushie or liquid form, this bubble tea will leave you energized and satisfied for the others of your entire day.

Chocolate (Preferably with Cheese Foam)

Who could say no to chocolate? If you're craving a liquid brownie, then you've found your match. While it's unique of hot chocolate, it still has that creamy, milky experience you might be heading for; if you manage to look for a shop that provides cream cheese foam, your tea will taste exactly like chocolate cheesecake. It's perfect as an after-dinner drink or dessert.

Passion fruit

An underrated flavour, passion fruit brings the tang most of us needed the bubble tea game. Another bubble tea flavor to consider the mouth area on an island getaway.

Fruity and vibrant, this flavor is guaranteed to wake your tastebuds perfectly.

Jasmine

Flowery, herbal, and mildly sweet? Jasmine may be the perfect option for all those buying more robust tea flavor. Quite often, you can find variations such as Jasmine green tea extract, which is simply as unusual, a little lighter. That one is actually for the tea lovers available.

Matcha

This delicious drink brings all of the health advantages of Japanese-style green tea extract using the texture of bubble tea. Matcha is usually another Asian flavour that has climbed; it's way up in popularity all over the world. It's a robust and herbal tea flavour that will please even the most distinguished palate.

Didn't enjoy it, to begin with? Bubble tea could be manufactured in many various ways with different ingredients, so that it may differ from spot to place. The next time you're in the mood for a new adventure, get one of these different places, an alternative flavour, various toppings, or ask to eliminate the tapioca pearls if that's what's off-putting. Everyone deserves to see the rich, deliciousness of milk tea, bubbles, or not.

Bubble tea could be a pretty daunting food to try; in the end, there's nothing else to enjoy it.

www.ingramcontent.com/pod-product-compliance
Lightning Source LLC
Chambersburg PA
CBHW071704210326
41597CB00017B/2330